PATIENT'S GUIDE TO RETINAL GENE THERAPY

Jeffrey N. Weiss, M.D.

Copyright (c) 2014 Jeffrey N. Weiss, M.D.

FOR ALL OUR PATIENTS

WHY DID I WRITE THIS BOOK?

I am the Principal Investigator of a study performing surgery for untreatable retinal and optic nerve conditions. When performing a new surgery for an untreatable condition, it is very important for the patient to fully understand the possible benefits and the risks of the procedure.

While it may be presumptuous to say, patient's participating in such a study always have a choice. That choice is to participate or not to participate. When patients come to my office, I always conclude my explanation of the surgery with the statement, "If you have any misgivings with what I have told you, then do not undergo the procedure. I would rather we part as friends then perform a procedure when you have reservations."

Patients sometimes say to me "My doctor never heard of this work." I point to my 6 telephone lines on the telephone in my examination room and suggest they invite their doctor to call me for a personal explanation. My study is listed on the National Institute of Health (NIH) website. I am available by telephone and email for any questions.

While it is impossible for a physician to know everything, in order to hold himself out as an expert for his patients, he should have an open and inquiring mind.

I believe that it is critical for physicians and patients to approach gene therapy for retina disease fairly and scientifically. It is vital that the required tests be performed in the postoperative period and that patients adhere to follow up requirements for progress to be made.

WHO IS THIS BOOK FOR?

Typically, this book will be read by the family member or friend of a patient who is losing or has already lost their vision. The patient has often been to many specialists over the years and been told that there is nothing anyone can do to stop the loss, or try to return their lost vision. So, frequently they haven't been to an eye doctor for several years because they are so discouraged.

SECTION 1

WHAT IS RESEARCH?

Research is conducted to prove, or disapprove, a hypothesis. A procedure may be "proven" to work, but may not be commonly "accepted" by most physicians. Why?" Because the procedure may be difficult or too time consuming to perform, too expensive in terms of the learning, drugs or equipment required, or not paid for by insurance companies. Remember, insurance companies are in business to make money. They do not pay for any procedure that they consider experimental. Their definition of "experimental" is anything outside the mainstream. So anything new and not commonly performed is not normally covered.

The insurance company may ask for articles and papers and you may appeal their decision not to reimburse, but it is highly unlikely that they will pay for the treatment. I know this to be the case, having been through this process for my patients many times. Not one appeal was successful and at the end of multiple appeals, the insurance company simply quoted the patient's insurance policy, which stated that their contract doesn't pay for experimental procedures. The process is dressed in the guise of a fair and objective hearing, but is designed to waste your time, hoping the patient or physician will eventually give up and go away as the decision not to pay was already made prior to all the appeals.

WHO PAYS FOR "RESEARCH?"

Research is paid for by grants from the Government, from pharmaceutical and device companies, from Universities, private foundations, and by patients.

The pharmaceutical industry has a research and development budget nearly double that of the National Institutes of Health. Sounds good? Not really. In 1990, they spent 8.4 billion dollars on research, and 55.2 billion dollars in 2006, but fewer successful drugs have been introduced, and of those, 75% of them are similar to already existing drugs. Only 25% offer an improvement over existing medications.

Especially now, in this time of budgetary cutbacks, only a small minority of worthwhile research grants are ever funded by the government. When funds are so limited there is political pressure to only fund studies with a pressing social impact. It may take a researcher more than a year to write a research proposal. Frequently the research proposal includes the data showing that the research has already been done! The results prove the hypothesis and further funding is needed to continue the work. Everyone, including the government, likes to "pick a winner" and this is made possible by already performing the study you are asking for the money to perform!

WHAT IS BIAS?

Pharmaceutical companies pay physicians handsomely to participate in drug research. They may pay for each patient included in the study, offer grant money for physician "research," pay honoraria for the doctor to give lectures, and pay travel expenses. The physician himself may have been given or own stock in the company. The physician is supposed to list his "financial disclosures" when presenting a paper or giving a talk.

Listing financial support doesn't eliminate bias, it just makes everyone aware of potential bias. The pharmaceutical companies pay many physicians in this manner, much like large companies contribute to both political parties, so it is commonplace to see financial disclosures. A doctor receiving this type of support is less likely to say something bad about the drug, instrument, or study. Physicians are people too, and as such, have the same emotions as everyone else. There is altruism, generosity, compassion, as well as jealously, envy and stubbornness.

All research, and indeed all work, has some degree of bias. The physician earns money performing treatments, and of course he wants the treatments to be successful. That is just human nature.

WHAT IS THE ROLE OF THE FDA?

The Food and Drug Administration (FDA) mission is to regulate food, drugs and medical devices and not the practice of medicine.

Medical advances come in two basic ways:

1. Large pharmaceutical companies spend many years testing drugs,
and perform large studies costing many hundreds of millions of dollars. The costs are so high that only potential blockbuster drugs are allowed to run the gauntlet of clinical trials. This accounts for the decreasing number of truly new drugs to fight or prevent diseases, i.e. antibiotics and vaccines.

2. Physicians initially produce anecdotal reports but move at a much more rapid pace and self-correct via education and peer review.

For example, the FDA has assumed authority over all stem cell transplants, with few exemptions. This was accomplished in 2006 by changing one word. The original rule spoke to cells and tissue placed "into another human." The new rule was changed to "into a human" which now means that stem cells, even your own, are now regulated by the FDA as a drug.

The effect of this regulation has been to drive investment, companies, research and jobs out of the U.S. and to other countries with less onerous regulation.

Consequently, many of the gene studies now listed on the National Institutes of Health website, being performed in the U.S., involve proprietary products and are supported by companies. The exceptions are those studies supported by Universities, or by the National Eye Institute. Frequently, the study is conducted under the authority of an Institutional Review Board or IRB, which is a committee of physicians, experts and lay people which insure the ethical and safe treatment of patients, and the scientific merits and validity of the proposed study.

Physician sponsored studies tend to be more quick to respond to changes that might improve outcomes. For example, during the last 6 months our study has, in response to published articles and our own patient observation, made changes in our procedure and modified our surgical procedure.

SECTION 2

WHAT DOES THE DIFFERENT PHASES OF A STUDY MEAN?

Phase 1 - A new drug or treatment is given to a small group of people, for the first time, to evaluate its safety, determine a safe dosage and monitor for side effects.

Phase 2 - The drug or treatment is given to a larger group of people to determine effectiveness and safety.

Phase 3 - The drug or treatment is given to large groups of people to determine effectiveness and safety, and to compare it to other commonly used treatments and collect data.

Phase 4 - These are studies performed after the drug or treatment has been marketed. They are performed to determine the effectiveness in various populations and identify side effects observed with long-term use.

WHAT IS EVIDENCE BASED MEDICINE?

Evidence-based medicine is defined as "the conscientious, explicit and judicious use of current best evidence in making decisions about the care of individual patients."

The United States Preventive Services Task Force has rated evidence concerning the effectiveness of treatment.

Level 1 - Evidence obtained from a properly designed randomized controlled trial.

Level II-1 - Evidence obtained from well-designed controlled trials without randomization.

Level ll-2 - Evidence obtained from a well-designed case-control or cohort study, preferably from more than one center or research group.

Level ll-3 - Evidence obtained from multiple time series with or without the intervention. Dramatic results in uncontrolled trials may be considered as this level of evidence.

Level lll - Opinions or reports of respected authorities or expert committees.

HOW DOES THE EYE WORK?

RETINA

The eye is like a video camera. The cornea is the clear part of the eye, overlying the iris or colored part, which focuses light through the lens of the eye which further focuses the image onto the retina. The retina is like the film in the camera.

We can divide the retina into two parts, the macula, and the peripheral retina. The macula represents approximately 5% of the retinal area, and the peripheral retina the remaining 95%. The macula is considered the center of the retina, and is associated with central vision. It allows you see tiny detail, drive a car, recognize faces and read this book. The other 95% of the retina is the peripheral retina which gives us our side vision. It allows us to notice movement "out of the corner of our eye" and is useful when walking down a street or driving an automobile so we are aware and able to notice what is around us.

OPTIC NERVE

The light hitting the retina is processed by the retina and the electrical signals are sent via the optic nerve to the brain for interpretation. Anything that affects the visual pathway can affect the vision. If we think of the eye as a video camera, the optic nerve is the electric cord that runs from the camera to the video monitor, or the brain. If the camera works, but the electric cord is cut, you don't see a picture.

RETINAL SURGERY

Injections - Intraretinal/Subretinal - Prior to injecting cells into or under the retina, a vitrectomy is performed. In this procedure, small instruments are placed into the eye and the vitreous body, (the natural gel inside the eye) is removed and replaced with a clear liquid. This surgery has been performed since the 1980's. The surgeon then has access to inject cells into or under the retina.

In this book, we are confining ourselves to gene studies treating retinal conditions.

SECTION 3

"GENETIC" DEFINITIONS

DNA - DNA (deoxyribonucleic acid) is the hereditary material present in cells that contains the biologic instructions that allows an organism to develop, survive, and reproduce. Most DNA is found inside the nucleus of the cell and is called nuclear DNA. A small portion of DNA is also found in small structures within the cell called mitochondria. The mitochondria generate the energy the cell uses to function. During human reproduction, the offspring inherits half of their nuclear DNA from the mother, and half from the father and all the mitochondrial DNA from the mother.

Genes – Genes are the basic unit of heredity consisting of a few hundred DNA bases to more than 2 million bases. These are the instructions by which we make molecules called proteins. 99% of all genes in all people are the same, less than 1% are different and it is this 1% that accounts for our differences. Humans have between 20,000 and 25,000 genes.

Chromosome - Each chromosome contains many genes. The DNA is tightly wrapped around proteins so they can fit inside the cell. If the DNA molecule in a single cell was unwound and placed end to end it would stretch 6 feet! A chromosome is a thread-like structure in the cell nucleus consisting of protein and DNA. For a person to grow and function properly, the cells must divide to make new cells and to replace old, worn-out cells. Chromosomes are important in ensuring that the DNA is correctly copied and distributed. As an example, patients with Downs Syndrome have 3 copies of chromosome 21, not the 2 copies found in other people. Humans have 46 chromosomes, half from the mother and half from the father, dogs have 39 chromosomes, and a fruit fly 4 chromosomes.

Human Genome Project - This was a 13 year long project that successfully identified and sequenced all the approximately 20,000 - 25,000 genes in human DNA.

Genome - A genome is all the DNA in an organism.

Locus - A position on a chromosome of a gene or other marker. The DNA at that position.

Autosomal - Refers to any of the chromosomes other than the X and Y chromosomes (the sex-determining chromosomes) or the genes on these chromosomes.

Autosomal dominant - Refers to one of several ways that a trait or disorder can be inherited. If a condition is autosomal dominant, it means you need the abnormal gene from one parent to inherit the condition.

Autosomal recessive - This means that two copies, one from each parent, of the abnormal gene must be present for you to inherit the condition

Allele - This word is a shortened version of the word "allelomorph" which was used in the early days of genetics to describe variant forms of a gene that can produce different observable phenotypic traits, such as different skin pigmentation.

"EYE" DEFINITIONS

Snellen visual acuity i.e. 20/20, etc. - In the U.S., the Snellen eye chart is placed at a standard distance of 20 feet. The 20/20 line is the smallest line that a person with normal acuity can read at 20 feet. For example, if a person can only read the line three lines above the 20/20 line, that is, the 20/40 line, that would be equivalent to what a normal person could read at 40 feet.

ETDRS visual acuity - This is an eye chart that is illuminated from behind so that the lighting is uniform and with the same number of letters on each line, that decrease in size, based on a mathematical formula. It was developed to provide a standardized way to measure visual acuity, which is important in the performance of clinical research studies.

Electroretinogram - This test measures the electrical responses of various cells in the retina. Electrodes are generally placed on the eye and the skin near the eye and the patient's eyes are exposed to flashing lights. The resulting signal is used in the diagnosis of various retinal diseases.

Optical Coherence Tomography (OCT) - OCT is a noninvasive test that uses light to make cross-sectional images of the retina and optic nerve. It allows the ophthalmologist to map and measure the thickness of the tissues.

"STUDY" DEFINITIONS

Autologous - Derived or transferred from the same individual's body. Also known as an "autograft" or "autotransplant."

Heterologous (Xenotransplant) - Derived or transferred from another species.

Homologous - Deriving from a common primitive origin.

Allograft - Tissue taken from an individual of the same species as the recipient but with different hereditary factors.

Open-label trial - Both patients and researcher know which treatment is being administered.

Single-blind trial - The patient does not know which treatment is being administered, but the researcher does.

Double-blind trial - Neither the patient nor the researcher knows what treatment is being administered.

Non-Randomized Trial - A clinical trial in which the participants choose which group they want to be in, or they are assigned to a particular treatment group by the researchers.

Randomized Trial - The participants are assigned by chance to different groups comparing different treatments. At the time of the trial, it is unknown which treatment is best. Neither the participants nor the researcher can choose the group.

Multi-Center Trial - A trial conducted at more than one center.

Incidence - A measure of the risk of developing a condition within a specified period of time.

Prevalence - The proportion of a population found to have a condition.

EYE CONDITIONS CAUSED BY GENETIC ABNORMALITIES

Genetic abnormalities have been implicated in more than 600 conditions affecting the eye. The following represent some of the most common conditions affecting the retina.

****
****
****

SECTION 4

CONDITIONS TREATED IN STUDIES

Leber congenital amaurosis (LCA)

This is a hereditary condition that leads to the loss of vision, often at an early age. The prevalence of LCA is 2 - 3 per 100,000 births. It comprises more than 5% of all retinal dystrophies and is the most common cause of inherited blindness in childhood. More than 20% of children attending schools for the blind have this condition. Some cases of LCA progress with time, others stabilize with time. At the present time 19 gene mutations have been identified which lead to different types of LCA.

Leber hereditary optic neuropathy (LHON)

This condition usually begins in a person's teens or twenties. Males are affected more often than females. Vision problems may begin in one eye, followed by the other eye in several weeks or months. Vision loss is characteristic of this condition though some patients may experience tremors, heart conduction defects and others develop symptoms similar to multiple sclerosis. LHON results from mutations in the cell's mitochondria or energy producing structure which are inherited from the mother through the eggs she produces. It has been associated with 4 gene mutations in the mitochondria of the egg cells that are passed to their offspring.

Achromatopsia

This condition is non-progressive and is characterized by decreased vision, light sensitivity and the absence of color vision. It is sometimes called "day blindness" because patients with this condition may see better in low light. Those with complete achromatopsia may see 20/200 or less, those patients with incomplete achromatopsia may see 20/80 - 20/120. At this time, 4 genes have been found to be associated with this condition.

Age-related Macular Degeneration (AMD)

AMD is a degenerative retinal disease related to age which generally begins when patients are in their 50's or early 60's and can lead to the loss of central vision. It is the leading cause of visual loss in this age group and older. AMD is typically divided into a "wet" or neovascular type and a "dry" type of AMD. The dry type may be further subdivided into typical dry AMD which may transition into the wet type and geographic atrophy. 88% of patients have the dry type and 12% the wet type of AMD, yet the wet type accounts for approximately 90% of the overall visual loss experienced by patients.

The wet type of AMD is characterized by the growth of new blood vessels under the retina, at or near the macula. These new blood vessels can leak fluid or blood leading to the loss of central vision and scarring. Injections of medicine and/or laser treatment are used to treat this condition.

Vitamins as recommended by the Age-related Eye Disease Study (AREDS) group can slow the progression of dry to wet AMD. At the present time, there is no treatment for geographic atrophy. This type of dry AMD is characterized by retinal atrophy which may be at, or around the center of vision. Patients with this condition may experience a loss of central vision or "holes" in their vision around their central vision.

Choroideremia

This condition mainly affects males and is characterized by progressive vision loss with the loss of night vision occurring in childhood. Progression of the condition varies, but generally leads to blindness in late adulthood. The prevalence of this condition is 1 in 50,000 - 100,000 people and accounts for 4% of all blindness. Choroideremia is inherited in an X-linked recessive pattern and has been ascribed to a mutation in the CHM gene. Males, who only have one X chromosome, (unlike females, which have 2 X chromosomes) are more affected by X-linked recessive disorders. If a female has one mutated copy of the gene on one of her X chromosomes, she is called a carrier of the condition. She may have no signs or symptoms of the condition, but can pass the mutated gene on to her offspring.

Cone dystrophy

This is an inherited or genetic condition in which the cone system is predominantly affected, although the rod system may be later affected. Most cases are of autosomal dominant inheritance. Age of onset, rate of progression and severity vary. The condition may begin in childhood, midlife, or at an older age. The progression of the loss of vision is more rapid in patients with the early onset of visual symptoms. The loss of vision may not be symmetric and is seldom much below 20/200. There is no treatment at the present time.

Cone-Rod Dystrophy

Patients with this condition generally present with a loss in central and color vision and the development of night blindness. The symptoms may start early in life or even in adulthood. This condition, also termed inverse pigmentary retinal dystrophy, may be related to retinitis pigmentosa.

Gyrate Atrophy

This condition is caused by a mutation in the OAT gene, which provides for an enzyme called ornithine ketoacid aminotransferase. The severity of symptoms is dependent on the type of mutation. Patients with this condition began experiencing night blindness, a decrease in the peripheral vision and nearsightedness. These progressive changes can lead to blindness at 50 years of age. Of the 150 patients identified with this condition, approximately 1/3 are from Finland.

Retinitis Pigmentosa (rod-cone dystrophies)

These terms refer to a large spectrum of retinal disorders of variable age of onset, progression rate, severity and mode of inheritance.

Patients with this condition typically experience a loss of night vision in childhood or early adulthood. There is a progressive contraction of the visual field and frequently profound loss of vision in middle or later life. Usher's Syndrome is typical retinitis pigmentosa with congenital deafness. The condition may be inherited or mutational.

There are related conditions, which may represent incomplete form of RP called atypical pigmentary retinal dystrophy's which are further subdivided into different conditions.

Stargardt's Macular Dystrophy

This is the most common juvenile retinal degenerative disease. Patients present with visual loss during childhood or early adulthood, although some experience symptoms later in life. It is inherited as an autosomal recessive trait in most patients.

Usher's Syndrome

This is the most common condition that affects both hearing and vision. The symptoms are hearing loss and retinitis pigmentosa. There are three types of Usher's syndrome, type 1, type 2, and type 3. Types 1 and 2 account for up to 95% of children who have this condition. It is inherited as an autosomal recessive trait.

Type 1 - Profound deafness from birth, decreased night vision before 10 years of age, balance problems from birth

Type 2 - Moderate to severe hearing loss from birth, decreased night vision beginning in late childhood or teens, normal balance

Type 3 - Normal hearing at birth, progressive loss of hearing in childhood or early teens, night vision problem often starting in the teenage years, normal to near-normal balance, with problems possibly starting later in life

****
****
****

SECTION 5

CLINICALTRIALS.GOV registered studies (NATIONAL INSTITUTES OF HEALTH (NIH) WEBSITE)

Information Current as of 1/17/14

"EYE GENE RETINA" LISTING

Note: The order of the listed studies is as appears on the NIH website. A lower numbered study is not meant to imply that it is somehow better than a higher numbered study. The number in parenthesis represents the study number as shown on the website. I have included only studies with active recruitment. The study order number is nonsequential because other non-retinal gene studies, as well as completed studies are also listed. The following information is taken from the NIH website from sites identified by typing "Eye Gene Retina" in the Search box. Not all studies have supplied all the information. I have, in some cases, simplified the information they provided and in other cases corrected contradictory information and spelling mistakes. I have done my best in representing the material that was provided in the "Full Text View" section of each study.

****
****
****
****
****

1. (1) TITLE - Trial of Ocular Subretinal Injection of a Recombinant Adeno-Associated Virus (rAAV2-VMD2-hMERTK) Gene Vector to Patients with Retinal Disease Due to MERTK Mutations

ClinicalTrials.gov Identifier: NCT01482195

OFFICIAL TITLE - Phase 1 Trial of Ocular Subretinal Injection of a

Recombinant Adeno-Associated Virus (rAAV2-VMD2-hMERTK) Gene Vector to Patients With Retinal Disease Due to MERTK Mutations

SPONSOR - Fowzan Alkuraya

COLLABORATORS

- King Khaled Eye Specialist Hospital

- King Faisal Specialist Hospital & Research Center

PURPOSE OF STUDY -

A recombinant adeno-associated virus serotype 2 (rAAV2) vector has been altered to carry the human MERTK (hMERTK) gene. This vector has been shown to restore vision in animal models that resemble human MERTK-associated Retinitis Pigmentosa (RP), an incurable retinal degeneration that causes severe vision loss. The proposed study is an open label, Phase I clinical trial of subretinal rAAV2-VMD2-hMERTK administration to individuals with MERTK-associated retinal disease. This trial will lead to a greater understanding of the safety and thereby potential value of gene transfer in MERTK-associated retinal disease and will have implications for other forms of retinal degenerative disease amenable to this type of intervention.

TYPE OF STUDY - Interventional

NUMBER OF PATIENTS TO BE ENROLLED - 6

STUDY SITE - King Khaled Eye Specialist Hospital, Riyadh, Saudi Arabia

PRINCIPAL INVESTIGATOR - Emad Abboud, M.D.

CONTACT - Deepak Edward, M.D. 966-1482-1234 ext. 1362
dedward@kkesh.med.sa

LENGTH OF STUDY - START DATE - August 2011
                    - END DATE - August 2023

PROCEDURE - Ocular Subretinal Injection of a Recombinant Adeno-Associated Virus

DETAILED DESCRIPTION - Not Supplied

****

2. (2) TITLE - Phase 1 Trial of Gene Vector to Patients with Retinal Disease Due to RPE65 Mutations (LCA)

ClinicalTrials.gov Identifier: NCT00481546

OFFICIAL TITLE - Phase 1 Trial of Ocular Subretinal Injection of a Recombinant Adeno-Associated Virus (RAAV2-CBSB-hRPE65) Gene Vector to Patients With Retinal Disease Due to REP65 Mutations (Clinical Trials of Gene Therapy for Leber Congenital Amaurosis).

SPONSOR - University of Pennsylvania

COLLABORATOR - National Eye Institute (NEI)

PURPOSE OF STUDY -

A recombinant adeno-associated virus serotype 2 (rAAV2) vector has been altered to carry the human RPE65 (hRPE65) gene. This vector has been shown to restore vision in animal models that resemble human RPE65-associated Leber congenital amaurosis (LCA), an incurable retinal degeneration that causes severe vision loss. The proposed study is an open label, Phase I clinical trial of subretinal rAAV2-CBSB-hRPE65 administration to individuals with RPE65-associated retinal disease. Five cohorts will be included in this trial. Cohorts 1, 2 and 4 will consist of individuals 18 years of age and older. Cohorts 3 and 5 will consist of individuals between the ages of 8 and 17, inclusive. Enrollment in Cohorts 3 and 5 will begin only after confirming the safety of rAAV2-CBSB-hRPE65 administration in the older groups of participants. This trial will lead to a greater understanding of the safety and thereby potential value of gene transfer in RPE65-associated retinal disease and will have implications for other forms of retinal degenerative disease amenable to this type of intervention.

The goal of this clinical trial is to determine the safety of uniocular subretinal administration of rAAV2-CBSB-hRPE65 in individuals with RPE65-associated retinal disease. Ocular and systemic toxicity will be assessed prior to and following vector administration to determine if there are adverse changes that may be associated with vector administration.

TYPE OF STUDY - Interventional

NUMBER OF PATIENTS TO BE ENROLLED - 15

STUDY SITES -

Shands Children's Hospital, University of Florida, Gainesville, Florida

Principal Investigator - Barry J. Byrne, MD, PhD
Contact: Sharon Wolfe-Schwartz, MS, CGC 215-662-9981
chrd@uphs.upenn.edu

Scheie Eye Institute, University of Pennsylvania, Philadelphia, Pennsylvania
Principal Investigator - Samuel G. Jacobson, MD, PhD
Contact: Sharon Wolfe-Schwartz, MS, CGC 215-662-9981
chrd@uphs.upenn.edu

LENGTH OF STUDY - START DATE - July 2007
- END DATE - June 2026

PROCEDURE - Not Provided

DETAILED DESCRIPTION - Not Provided

****
****
****

3. (6) TITLE - Gene Therapy for Blindness Caused by Choroideremia

ClinicalTrial. gov Identifier NCT01461213

OFFICIAL TITLE - An Open Label Dose Escalation Phase 1 Clinical Trial of Retinal Gene therapy For Choroideremia Using an Adeno-associated Viral Vector(AAV2) Encoding Rab-escort Protein 1 (REP1)

SPONSOR

University of Oxford

COLLABORATORS

Oxford University Hospitals NHS Trust
Moorfields Eye Hospital NHS Foundation Trust
University College, London
Central Manchester University Hospitals NHS Foundation Trust
University of Manchester
University Hospital Southampton NHS Foundation Trust
University of Southampton

PURPOSE OF STUDY -

To assess the safety and tolerability of the AAV.REP1 vector, administered at two different doses to the retina in 12 patients with a diagnosis of choroideremia.

To identify any therapeutic benefit as evidenced by a slowing down of the retinal degeneration assessed by functional and anatomical methods in the treated eye compared to the control eye 24 months after gene delivery.

TYPE OF STUDY - Interventional

NUMBER OF PATIENTS TO BE ENROLLED - 12

STUDY SITES

Moorfields Eye Hospital NHS Foundation Trust, London, United Kingdom
Principal Investigator, Andrew R. Webster
Contact 020 7566 2260
St. Mary's Hospital, Central Manchester University Hospitals NHS Foundation Trust, Manchester, United Kingdom
Principal Investigator, Graeme C. Black
Contact 0161 276 6269

Oxford Radcliffe Hospitals NHS Trust, Oxford, United Kingdom
Principal Investigator, Susan Downes
Contact 01865 231578

Eye Unit, Southampton University Hospitals NHS Trust, Southamptom, United Kingdom
Principal Investigator, Andrew J. Lotery
Contact 023 8079 4590

INVESTIGATORS

Study Chair - Robert E. MacLaren, MB, ChB, DPhil
University of Oxford, Oxford Radcliffe Hospitals NHS Trust and Moorfields Eye Hospital

Principal Investigator - Miguiel C. Seabra, MD, PhD
Imperial College, London

Principal Investigator - Andrew R. Webster, MD UCL Institute of Ophthalmology and Moorfields Eye Hospital

Principal Investigator - Susan M. Downes, MD Oxford University Hospitals NHS Trust

Principal Investigator - Graeme C. Black, MB, BCh, DPhil University of Manchester and Central Manchester University Hospitals NHS Foundation Trust

Principal Investigator - Andrew J. Lotery, MD University of Southampton and Southampton University Hospitals Trust

Principal Investigator - Len W. Seymour, PhD University of Oxford
Principal Investigator - Tanya Tolmachova, PhD Imperial College London

LENGTH OF STUDY - START DATE - October 2011

- END DATE - June 2016

PROCEDURE

Arm 1 - Single subretinal injection of up to 10e 10 genome particles

Arm 2 - Single subretinal injection of up to 10e 11 genome particles

DETAILED DESCRIPTION - Not Provided

****

4. (7) TITLE - Safety and Efficacy Study in Subjects With Leber Congenital Amaurosis

ClinicalTrial.gov Identifier - NCT000999609

OFFICIAL TITLE - A Safety and Efficacy Study in Subjects With Leber Congenital Amaurosis (LCA) Using Adeno-Associated Viral Vector to Deliver the Gene for Human RPE65 to the Retinal Pigment Epithelium (RPE) [AAV2-hRPE65v2-301]

SPONSOR - Spark Therapeutics, LLC

COLLABORATORS -

Children's Hospital of Philadelphia

University of Iowa

PURPOSE OF STUDY -

The study is a Phase 3, open-label, randomized controlled trial of gene therapy intervention by subretinal administration of AAV2-hRPE65v2. At least twenty-four subjects, three years of age or older, will be recruited. The intervention group will receive AAV2-hRPE65v2 vector at either The Children's Hospital of Philadelphia, or University of Iowa to determine if it improves visual and retinal function in individuals with LCA2.

TYPE OF STUDY - Interventional

NUMBER OF PATIENTS TO BE ENROLLED - 24

STUDY SITES -

University of Iowa, Iowa City, Iowa
Principal Investigator - Stephen R. Russell, MD
Contact - Jean Walshire   jean-walshire@uiowa.edu

Children's Hospital of Philadelphia, Philadelphia, Pennsylvania
Principal Investigator - Albert M. Maguire, MD
Contact - Kathleen Marshall
marshallk1@email.chop.edu
Contact - Dominique Cross, MS
crossd2@email.chop.edu

LENGTH OF STUDY - START DATE - OCTOBER 2012
                - END DATE - April 2029 (?)

PROCEDURE - Not Provided

DETAILED DESCRIPTION -

Leber congenital amaurosis (LCA) is a disease where part of the eye (the retina) is severely diseased. Usually it is detected in affected people within the first few months of life, as there is significantly poor vision at birth. Cells in the retina are lost over time in people with LCA which leads to total blindness. There are no pharmacological treatments available. This study will focus on the form of LCA caused by changes (mutations) in DNA that make a certain protein (called in 65 kDa retinal pigment epithelium (RPE)-specific protein, or RPE65). Clinical diagnosis is made by function tests of the eye. This can be confirmed by a special method of testing (molecular testing) to verify that the RPE65 is not correct.

This study uses a gene therapy vector made from an adeno-associated virus (AAV) called AAV2-hRPE65v2. Gene therapy refers to the incorporation of new DNA into cells with the goal of supplying a therapeutic gene or a gene that is missing or not functioning in the cell. The AAV parts of the gene therapy vector work as a delivery vehicle for getting the normal human RPE65 gene into the cells of the retina. An earlier clinical study of AAV2-

hRPE65v2 was conducted based on the demonstration of safety and effectiveness of the vector in animals with a similar eye disease. The earlier clinical study tested three doses of the vector in twelve children and adults. The three doses were safe for the eye and the rest of the body in individuals as young as eight years old. AAV2-hRPE65v2 administration also led to increased vision in the subjects, with the youngest subjects showing the most improvement.

The study will deliver AAV2-hRPE65v2 vector to at least sixteen intervention group subjects, age three or older, subjects will receive the vector in both eyes via subretinal injections during surgeries (on separate days). The purpose of this research study is to assess the effectiveness and safety of the AAV2-hRPE65v2 gene therapy vector as a possible treatment for LCA2. The control group of at least eight subjects will be able to cross-over to the intervention group after one year, provided they still meet all eligibility criteria.

****

5. (10) TITLE - Clinical Trial of Gene Therapy for Leber Congenital Amaurosis Caused by RPE65 Mutations

ClinicalTrials.gov Identifier - NCT00821340

OFFICIAL TITLE - Phase 1 Trial of Ocular Subretinal Injection of a Recombinant Adeno-Associated Virus (rAAV2-hRPE65) Gene Vector to Patients with Retinal Disease Due to RPE65 Mutations

SPONSOR - Hadassah Medical Organization

PURPOSE -

The purpose of this clinical trial is to examine the safety of gene therapy for Lebers Congenital Amaurosis (LCA) caused by RPE65 mutations using a recombinant adeno-associated virus serotype 2(rAAV2) vector carrying the human RPE65 (hRPE65) gene. Recently, three independent short-term gene therapy studies in humans with LCA due to RPE65 mutations were published, suggesting that subretinal delivery of rAAV virus carrying the RPE65 gene is safe. As a secondary outcome, improvement in visual function was observed in seven of the first nine treated patients. The proposed study is a similar open label, Phase I clinical trial of uniocular subretinal rAAV2-hRPE65 administration to individuals with RPE65-

associated retinal disease. Two cohorts of three subjects each and one cohort of four subjects will be included in this trial. Cohort 1 and 2 will consist of individuals 18 years of age and older and Cohorts 3 will consist of individuals 8 years of age and older. In cohort 2, a larger volume of vector will be administered. Enrollment in Cohort 3 will begin only after confirming the safety of rAAV2-hRPE65 administration in the older group of participants.

TYPE OF STUDY - Interventional

NUMBER OF PATIENTS TO BE ENROLLED - 10

STUDY SITE -

Hadassah Medical Organization, Jerusalem, Israel
Principal Investigator - Euyal Banin, MD, PhD

Contact - Devora Marks Ohana 00 972 2 6776324 devoramarks@gmail.com

LENGTH OF STUDY - START DATE - January 2010
- END DATE - January 2017

PROCEDURE - Not Provided

DETAILED DESCRIPTION - Not Provided

****

6. (12). TITLE Safety and Efficacy Study of rAAV.sFlt-1 in Patients With Exudative Age-related Macular Degeneration (AMD)

ClinicalTrials.gov Identifier
NCT01494805

OFFICIAL TITLE - A Phase 1/2 Controlled Dose-escalating Trial to Establish the Baseline Safety and Efficacy of a Single Subretinal Injection of rAAV.sFlt-1 Into Eyes of Patients With exudative Age-related Macular Degeneration (AMD)

SPONSOR - Lions Eye Institute, Perth, Western Australia

COLLABORATOR - Avalanche Biotechnologies, Inc.

PURPOSE OF STUDY -

The study will involve 48 patients aged 55 and above who have exudative age-related macular degeneration (wet AMD). Patients will be randomized to receive one of two doses of rAAV.sFlt-1 or assigned to the control group.

TYPE OF STUDY - Interventional

NUMBER OF PATIENTS TO BE ENROLLED - 48

STUDY SITE -

Lions Eye Institute, Perth, Western Australia
Principal Investigator - Professor Ian Constable, Lions Eye Institute
Contact - Cora Pierce, RN +61 8 9381 0750 corapierce@lei.org.au
Contact - Clinical Network Services +61(0)7 3719 6000 cns@clinical.net.au

LENGTH OF STUDY - START DATE - December 2011

- END DATE -

December 2016

PROCEDURE - Not Provided

DETAILED DESCRIPTION -

A new treatment for exudative age-related macular degeneration (wet AMD) is being investigated. The purpose of the Phase 1/2 clinical research study is to examine the baseline safety and efficacy of an experimental study drug to treat a complication of the disease which leads to vision loss. The name of the study drug is rAAV.sFlt-1.

This experimental study uses a non-pathogenic virus to express a therapeutic protein within the eye. The therapeutic diminishes the growth of abnormal blood vessels under the retina. The duration of effect is thought to be long-term (years) following a single administration.

The clinical research study will look at the baseline safety and efficacy of a single injection of rAAV.sFlt-1 injected directly into the eye.

Forty-eight (48) patients will participate in Australia. The primary endpoint of the study is at one month, with extended follow up for 3 years.

****

7. (36) TITLE - PHASE 1/2a Study of StarGen in Patients With Stargardt Macular Degeneration

ClinicalTrials.gov Identifier - NCT01367444

OFFICIAL TITLE - A Phase 1/2a Dose Escalation Safety Study of Subretinally Injected StarGen Administered to Patients With Stargardt Macular Degeneration

SPONSOR - Oxford BioMedica

PURPOSE OF STUDY -

The purpose of this first in man study is to examine the safety of an experimental gene transfer agent, StarGen, designed to treat Stargardt Macular Degeneration.

TYPE OF STUDY - Interventional

NUMBER OF PATIENTS TO BE ENROLLED - 28

STUDY SITES -

Casey Eye Institute, Oregon Health & Science University, Portland, Oregon

Principal Investigator - David Wilson, MD

Hospitalier Nationale d'Ophthalmologie des Quinze-Vingts, Paris, France
Principal Investigator - Jose Sahel, MD, PhD
Contact - Jose Sahel, MD, PhD

LENGTH OF STUDY - START DATE - June 2011
 - END DATE - October 2013 (Still listed as recruiting participants as of 1/17/14.)

PROCEDURE - Not Provided

DETAILED DESCRIPTION -

There are two parts to the study. A dose-escalation phase looking at three doses of StarGen, eight patients will be recruited at the first dose level, and four each at the next two dose levels. This will be followed by a dose confirmation phase where the highest dose that is safe and well tolerated will be examined in up to twelve patients.

****

8. (47) TITLE - Study of UshStat in Patients With Retinitis Pigmentosa Associated With Usher Syndrome Type 1B

ClinicalTrials.gov Identifier - NCT01505062

OFFICIAL TITLE - A Phase 1/2a Dose Escalation Safety Study of Subretinally Injected UshStat, Administered to Patients With Retinitis Pigmentosa Associated With Usher Syndrome Type 1B

SPONSOR - Oxford BioMedica

PURPOSE OF STUDY -

The purpose of this first in man study is to examine the safety of an experimental gene transfer agent, UshStat designed to treat retinitis pigmentosa associated with Usher Syndrome Type 1B

STUDY TYPE - Interventional

NUMBER OF PATIENTS TO BE ENROLLED - 18

STUDY SITES -

Casey Eye Institute, Oregon Health & Science University, Portland, Oregon
Principal Investigator - Richard G. Weleber, MD
Hospitalier Nationale d'Ophthalmologie des Quinze-Vingts, Paris, France

Principal Investigator - Jose-Alain Sahel, MD, PhD

LENGTH OF STUDY - START DATE - January 2012
                    - END DATE - December 2014

DETAILED DESCRIPTION -

Following screening procedures the gene transfer agent will be injected once only under one retina by an ophthalmic surgeon under anesthesia. Patients will then have regular follow up visits where general health examinations, blood tests and ophthalmic examinations including best corrected visual acuity, slit lamp examination, intraocular pressure, fundoscopy, autofluorescence, Optical Coherence Tomography, perimetry and Electroretinogram will be undertaken.

****
****
****

9. (76) TITLE - Phase 1 Dose Escalation Safety Study of RetinoStat in Advanced Age-related Macular Degeneration (AMD)

ClinicalTrials.gov Identifier - NCT01301443

OFFICIAL TITLE - A Phase 1 Dose Escalation SafetyStudy of Subretinally Injected RetinoStat, a Lentiviral Vector Expressing Endostatin and Angiostatin, in Patients With Advanced Neovascular Age-related Macular Degeneration

SPONSOR - Oxford BioMedica

PURPOSE OF STUDY -

The purpose of this first in man study is to examine the safety of an experimental gene transfer agent, RetinoStat, designed to treat neovascular Age-related Macular Degeneration.
TYPE OF STUDY - Interventional

NUMBER OF PATIENTS TO BE ENROLLED - 18

STUDY SITES -

Johns Hopkins University Hospital, Baltimore, Maryland
Principal Investigator - Peter Campochiaro, MD

Andreas Lauer, MD, Portland, Oregon
Principal Investigator - Andreas Lauer, MD

LENGTH OF STUDY - START DATE - February 2011

- END DATE -

March 2014

DETAILED DESCRIPTION -

There are two parts to the study. A dose-escalation phase looking at three doses of RetinoStat starting with the lowest dose, three patients will be recruited at each dose level. The escalation phase will be followed by a dose confirmation phase where the highest dose that is safe and well tolerated will be examined in 9 patients.

****
****
****************styled

10. (77) TITLE - A Study to Determine the Long Term Safety, Tolerability and Biological Activity of

StarGen in Patients with Stargardt's Macular Degeneration

ClinicalTrials.gov Identifier - NCT01736592

OFFICIAL TITLE - An Open Label Study to Determine the Long Term Safety, Tolerability and Biological Activity of StarGen in Patients with Stargardt's Macular Degeneration

SPONSOR - Oxford BioMedica

PURPOSE OF STUDY - The purpose of the study is to examine the long term safety of an experimental gene transfer agent, StarGen, designed to treat Stargardt's Macular Degeneration.

STUDY TYPE - Interventional

NUMBER OF PATIENTS TO BE ENROLLED - 28 (ENROLLING BY INVITATION ONLY)

STUDY SITES -

Oregon Health and Science University, Portland, Oregon
Principal Investigator - David Wilson, MD

Centre National d'Ophtalmologie des Quinze-Vingts, Paris, France
Principal Investigator - Jose-Alain Sahel, MD

LENGTH OF STUDY - START DATE - December 2012
- END DATE - November 2028 (?)

DETAILED DESCRIPTION - Not Provided

Note - Uses LentiVector technology which is a "stripped-down" version of the equine infectious anemia virus (EIAV) to deliver a corrected version of the ABCR gene.

****

11. (78) TITLE - A Follow-up Study to Evaluate the Safety of RetinoStat in Patients with Age-Related Macular Degeneration

ClinicalTrials.gov Identifier - NCT01678872

OFFICIAL TITLE - A Long Term Follow-up Study to Evaluate the Safety of RetinoStat in Patients With Age-related Macular Degeneration

SPONSOR - Oxford BioMedica

PURPOSE -

The purpose of this study is to examine the long term safety of an experimental gene transfer agent, RetinoStat, designed to treat neovascular age-related macular degeneration.

STUDY TYPE - Interventional

NUMBER OF PATIENTS TO BE ENROLLED - 18 (ENROLLMENT BY INVITATION ONLY)

STUDY SITE -

Johns Hopkins University Hospital, Baltimore, Maryland
Principal Investigator - Peter Campochiaro, MD

LENGTH OF STUDY - START DATE - August 2012   - END DATE - November 2027

DETAILED DESCRIPTION - Not Provided

****
****
****
****
****

CLINICALTRIALS.GOV registered studies (NATIONAL INSTITUTES OF HEALTH (NIH) WEBSITE)

Information Current as of 1/17/14

"EYE GENE SURGERY" LISTING

Note: The order of the listed studies is as appears on the NIH website. A lower numbered study is not meant to imply that it is somehow better than a higher numbered study. The number in parenthesis represents the study number as shown on the website. The order is nonsequential because other non-retinal gene studies are also listed. In this section I have included also included some interesting "completed" and "active but not recruiting" studies.

The following information is taken from the NIH website from sites identified by typing "Eye Gene Surgery" in the Search box. Not all studies have supplied all the information. I have, in some cases, simplified the information they provided and in other cases corrected contradictory information and spelling mistakes. I have done my best in representing the material that was provided in the "Full Text View" section of each study.

****
****

1. (3) TITLE - Gene Therapy for Gyrate Atrophy

ClinicalTrials.gov Identifier: NCT00001735

OFFICIAL TITLE - Phase 1 Study in the Safety and Efficacy of Transduced Keratinocytes for Possible Treatment of Gyrate Atrophy.

SPONSOR - National Eye Institute

PURPOSE OF STUDY -

To evaluate the safety and effectiveness of gene therapy for patients with gyrate atrophy. Currently, this condition is treated with amino acid tablets and a very low-protein diet with limited fruits and vegetables and more than 2,000 calories a day from carbohydrates and fats. This is a difficult diet to follow and another alternative is to replace the defective gene with one that functions normally.

TYPE OF STUDY - Interventional

NUMBER OF PATIENTS TO BE ENROLLED - 5

STUDY SITE - National Eye Institute, Bethesda, Maryland

PRINCIPAL INVESTIGATOR - Not Listed

CONTACT - Not Listed

LENGTH OF STUDY - START DATE - April 1998

- END DATE - October 2000 (Completed - interesting work)

PROCEDURE -

Study patients will undergo the following gene therapy procedure:

1. Skin biopsy - A small piece of skin is surgically removed from the patient's thigh.

2. Gene transfer - Skin cells call keratinocytes are taken from the biopsied tissue and grown in the laboratory. The normal gene that produces the enzyme, ornithine aminotransferase (OAT) is inserted into

the cells, causing them to produce more of the enzyme.

3. Skin graft - Under local anesthesia, a patch of skin about 2 1/4 inches x 2 1/4 inches is surgically removed from the upper thigh and some of the cells with increased OAT are grafted back onto this area.

DETAILED DESCRIPTION -

The purpose of this phase 1 study is to evaluate the safety of a skin engraftment procedure for transplanting transduced keratinocytes in patients with a deficiency of the gene, OAT. The safety of this procedure will be evaluated in terms of technical complications and immune response of the patient. Keratinocytes, previously obtained and grown in culture from these patients, will be transduced with a retrovirus to express the OAT gene. The autologous transduced keratinocytes will be returned to the patient. At study defined visits, biopsies of the grafted area will be performed. The three secondary study objectives are: 1. the ability of the keratinocytes to express the OAT gene, 2. the extent and duration of such expression, and 3. the extent to which the activity present in the keratinocytes is sufficient to lower serum levels of ornithine.

****
****
****

2. (4) TITLE - CNTF Implants for CNGB3 Achromatopsia

ClinicalTrials.gov Identifier: NCT0648452

OFFICIAL TITLE - A Phase 1/2 Study of the NT-501 Intraocular Releasing Ciliary Neurotrophic Factor (CNTF) in Participants with CNGB3 Achromatopsia

SPONSOR - National Eye Institute (NEI)

PURPOSE OF STUDY -

1. Achromatopsia is an inherited condition that causes visual loss, sensitivity to light, and loss of color vision. There are no effective treatments.

2. Four genes are known to cause achromatopsia. One of these, the CNGB gene, is the cause in about 50 percent of people.

3. CNTF is a natural chemical found in the body that promotes survival and function of nerve cells. CNTF has been shown to be effective in treating

retinal disease in animals and can slow vision loss.

4. CNTF has been studied in over 250 people with other retinal diseases. The studies suggest that a CNTF implant might help vision in some eye diseases.

TYPE OF STUDY - Interventional

NUMBER OF PATIENTS TO BE ENROLLED - 5

STUDY SITE - National Eye Institute, Bethesda, Maryland

CONTACT - Not Provided

LENGTH OF STUDY - START DATE - July 2012
- END DATE - March 2014 (Active study, but not recruiting patients as of 1/17/14)

PROCEDURE -

The study requires 11 visits to the NEI over 3 years. One visit will be for the implant surgery. The implant will be placed in one eye only. At the 3 year visit, you can choose to keep the CNTF implant in your eye, or you can have it removed.

DETAILED DESCRIPTION -

The objective of the study is to evaluate the safety of ocular NT-501 device with encapsulated NT-201 cells releasing Ciliary Neurotrophic Factor)CNTF) to the retina of participants affected with CNGB3 achromatopsia. One eye of each participant will receive a vitreous NT-501 device implant releasing CNTF. The study will be completed once the final participant has received three years of follow-up.

The primary outcome is the number and severity of adverse events and systemic and ocular toxicities at six months post-implantation. Assessment of retinal function, ocular structure and occurrence of adverse events will be performed. Secondary outcomes include changes in visual acuity and color vision, electroretinogram responses, and retinal imaging with optical coherence tomography.

****

3. (9) TITLE - Molecular Genetics of Retinal Degenerations

ClinicalTrials.gov identifier: NCT00231010

OFFICIAL TITLE - Molecular Genetics of Retinal Degenerations

SPONSOR - National Eye Institute (NEI)

PURPOSE OF STUDY -

This multinational study will investigate the inheritance of genetic retinal degeneration in families of different nationalities and ethnic backgrounds in order to identify the genes that, when altered, cause retinal degeneration. Patients with retinitis pigmentosa and closely related diseases such as Usher syndrome, snowflake vitreoretinal dystrophy and Bietti crystalline dystrophy may be eligible for this study.

TYPE OF STUDY - Observational

NUMBER OF PATIENTS TO BE ENROLLED - 5000

STUDY SITES -

1. University of California, San Diego

2. National Institutes of Health Clinical Center, Bethesda, Maryland
3. Harvard Medical School, Boston, Massachusetts

4. Cleveland Clinic Foundation, Children's Hospital, Cleveland, Ohio

5. Sun Yat-Sen University, Guangzhou, China

6. Aravind Eye Hospital, Maduri, India

7. University of Punjab, Lahore, Pakistan

PRINCIPAL INVESTIGATOR - James F. Hejtmancik, M.D., National Eye Institute

CONTACT - James F. Hejtmancik, M.D.
(301) 435-1598 f3h@helix.nih.gov

LENGTH OF STUDY - START DATE - September 2005
                    - END DATE - last update January 14, 2014

PROCEDURE -

1. Medical and surgical history

2. Examination to identify the type of retinal degeneration

3. Eye examination including tests of color vision, field of vision and night vision

4. Electroretinogram

5. Hearing test with a personal or family history of deafness

6. Balance testing, tests of coordination and caloric testing

7. Blood sample collection for genetic testing.

DETAILED DESCRIPTION -

This project will study the inheritance of genetic retinal degenerations in families of many nationalities and ethnic backgrounds in order to identify the genes that, when mutated, cause retinal degenerations and the pathophysiology through which they act.

Detailed examinations will be performed to characterize the patient's retinal degeneration and affectation status. A blood sample will be analyzed to identify the specific gene and the mutations that are associated with the retinal degeneration.

****
****
****

4. (11) TITLE - Safety and Efficacy Study in Subjects With Leber Congenital Amaurosis

ClinicalTrials.gov Identifier: NCT00999609

OFFICIAL TITLE - A Safety and Efficacy Study in Subjects With Leber Congenital Amaurosis (LCA) Using Adeno-Associated Viral Vector to Deliver the Gene for Human RPE65 to the Retinal Pigment Epithelium (RPE) [AAV2-hRPE65v2-301]

SPONSOR - Spark Therapeutics, LLC

COLLABORATORS -

Children's Hospital of Philadelphia

University of Iowa

PURPOSE OF STUDY -

The study is a Phase 3, open-label, randomized controlled trial of gene therapy intervention by subretinal administration of AAV2-hRPE65v2.

TYPE OF STUDY - Interventional

NUMBER OF PATIENTS TO BE ENROLLED - 24

STUDY SITES -

University of Iowa, Iowa City, Iowa
Contact - Jean Walshire   jean-walshire@uiowa.edu

Principal Investigator - Stephen R. Russell, M.D.

Children's Hospital of Philadelphia, Philadelphia, Pennsylvania
Contact - Kathleen Marshall
marshallk1@email.chop.edu
Contact - Dominique Cross, M.S.
crossd2@email.chop.edu
Principal Investigator - Albert M. Maguire, M.D.

LENGTH OF STUDY - START DATE - October 2012
- END DATE - April 2015

PROCEDURE -

Subretinal administration of gene therapy vector AAV2-hRPE65v2 (1.5E11 vector genomes per eye) to both eyes via surgical procedures on separate days.

DETAILED DESCRIPTION -

The study will focus on the form of LCA caused by mutations in DNA that makes a certain protein (called the 65 kDa retinal pigment epithelium specific protein or RPE65).

The study uses a gene therapy vector made from an adeno-associated virus (AAV) called AAV2-hRPE65v2. The AAV parts of the gene therapy vector work as a delivery vehicle for getting the normal RPE65 gene into the cells of the retina. The study will deliver the vector to at least 16 subjects, age 3 or older, subjects will receive the vector in both eyes via subretinal injections during surgeries performed on separate days. The purpose of this study is to assess the effectiveness and safety of the gene therapy vector as a possible treatment for LCA. The control group of at least eight subjects will be able to cross-over to the intervention group after one year, provided they still meet eligibility criteria.

Note - An earlier clinical study tested three doses of the vector in twelve children and adults. Administration led to an increased vision in the subjects, with the youngest subjects showing the most improvement.

****

5. (24) TITLE Studies of the Natural History and Pathogenesis and Outcome of Neonatal Onset Multisystem

Inflammatory Disease (NOMID/CAPS, DIRA,CRMO, Still's Disease, Behcet's Disease, and Other Undifferentiated Autoinflammatory Diseases).

ClinicalTrials.gov identifier: NCT00059748

OFFICIAL TITLE - Same as above

SPONSOR - National Institute of Arthritis and Musculoskeletal and Skin Diseases (NIAMS)

PURPOSE OF STUDY -

This study will examine and test patients with neonatal onset multi-system inflammatory disease (NOMID) to learn more about the cause and course of the disease. It will study the disease signs and symptoms and the possible role of a gene called CIAS1, and it will develop a database to gather information on patients with NOMID in the United States and around the world. It will also serve as a screening protocol to offer eligible patients participation in a treatment protocol, if an appropriate one is available.

Patients with this rare disease usually develop a chronic rash in the first days to weeks of life that can affect the entire body. Almost all patients have eye problems such as inflammation, optic atrophy, or swelling of the optic nerve. Joint problems can lead to sever disability. Nervous system problems can include chronic meningitis, brain atrophy, seizures, mental retardation, migraine headaches, hearing loss and others.

Patients with NOMID whose symptoms include a rash since birth along with one of the following: joint disease or bone overgrowth; central nervous system problem, eye problems, enlarged liver and spleen, or elevated inflammatory markers (substances that indicate inflammation) may be eligible for this study.

TYPE OF STUDY - Observational

NUMBER OF PATIENTS TO BE ENROLLED - Open

STUDY SITE - National Institutes of Health Clinical Center, Bethesda, Maryland

PRINCIPAL INVESTIGATOR - Raphaela Goldbach-Manskt, M.D.

CONTACT - Nicole Plass, R.N. (301) 496-2237 plassn@mail.nih.gov
         Raphaela Goldbach-Manskt, M.D. (301) 435-6243
goldbacr@mail.nih.gov

LENGTH OF STUDY - START DATE - April 2003
              - END DATE - Open

PROCEDURE -

Medical history and physical neurological, and eye examination

Hearing test

Completion of quality of life questionnaires

Evaluation of memory and learning ability
Urine test

Blood tests for genetic analysis, HIV infection, and other laboratory values

Blood test to evaluate growth hormones. (optional test)

Lumbar puncture (spinal tap) to collect cerebrospinal fluid (CSF) from the spinal canal

Skin biopsy to characterize the rash

Photographs of the patient to document the skin rash and joint changes

X-rays and magnetic resonance (MRI) scans of the knees or other affected joints

Brain MRI to evaluate central nervous system involvement, (if patient can lie still for 45 minutes)

Bone density scan to evaluate bone mineralization

DETAILED DESCRIPTION -

Autoinflammatory multisystem diseases are a group of diseases that are characterized by recurrent episodes of systemic inflammation as well as organ specific inflammation that can involve the skin, eyes, joints, bones, serosal surfaces, inner ear, and brain. The prominent role of IL-1 in the pathogenesis of these disorders has first become evident through the discovery of mutations in CIAS1 causing the cryopyrin-associated periodic syndromes (CAPS) including the most severe presentation Neonatal Onset Multisystem inflammatory Disease (NOMID).

We recently identified a new autoinflammatory disease DIRA (Deficiency of IL-1 Receptor Antagonist), a disease that is caused by mutations in IL1RN. Therapy with anakinra, the IL-1 receptor antagonist, can be life-saving. We also study additional rare diseases including CANDLE (chronic atypical neutrophilic dermatosis with lipodystrophy and elevated temperatures), the spectrum CRMO (Chronic Recurrent Multifocal Osteomyelitis). Still s disease, and Behcet's disease (BD) all of which may involve dysregulation of IL-1.

In this research protocol we seek to comprehensively evaluate affected patients clinically, genetically, immunologically, and endocrinologically. In addition, we intend to evaluate long term outcome and biomarkers. Eligibility for ongoing and planned treatment protocols will be determined by screening patients in this protocol. We plan to evaluate patients on a consultative basis for other autoinflammatory diseases for possible enrollment into this study.

****

6. (26) TITLE - Risk Factors for Drusen Progression

ClinicalTrials.gov Identifier:
NCT01830608

OFFICIAL TITLE - Same

SPONSOR - Medical University of Vienna

PURPOSE OF STUDY -

Age-related macular degeneration (AMD) is the leading cause of blindness in the Western World. The etiology and pathogenesis of this disease remain largely unknown. In Europe about two million people suffer from AMD.

According to the Age-Related Eye Disease Study (AREDS) the disease can be classified into early, intermediate and late.

Early age-related macular degeneration is characterized by the presence of small or medium-sized drusen and/or retinal pigmentary abnormalities.

Intermediate age-related macular degeneration is characterized by large drusen or numerous medium-size drusen and/or geographic atrophy not extending to the center of the macula.

Late age-related macular degeneration can be either atrophic with extension to the macula or neovascular. The late form of the disease is associated with a pronounced loss of visual acuity.

In the recent years several studies focused on risk factors for late AMD and a recent systematic review and meta-analysis reported risk factors for AMD based on 16 studies in almost 114,000 subjects. Strong and consistent associations with late AMD was found for increasing age, current cigarette smoking, previous cataract surgery, and a family history of AMD.

Consistent associations between late AMD and higher body mass index, history of cardiovascular disease, hypertension and higher plasma fibrinogen were also found, but association was weak. Inconsistent associations were found for gender ethnicity, diabetes, iris color, history of cerebrovascular disease, serum total and HDL cholesterol and triglyceride levels.

Evidence has also accumulated that other factors influence the risk for AMD. Several genetic risk factors have been identified in the last years including genes in the alternative complement pathway and the RMS2/HTRA1 region. In addition, post-hoc analysis of data from the AREDS study has indicated that reduced intake of the omega-3 free fatty acids eicosapentaenoic acid and docsahexaenoic acid are associated with the risk of late AMD thereby supporting previous population based studies. The AREDS study also revealed that reduced intake of the macular pigment lutein and zeaxanthin may be associated with late AMD, again supporting previous population-based studies. Finally, 2 small studies indicate that reduced choroidal blood flow is associated with an increased risk of developing late AMD.

Less data are available for the progression of early or intermediate AMD and the associated risk factors. This is at least partially related to the problems in quantifying progression of drusen size and volume. In the recent years, however, significant efforts have been achieved in optical coherence tomography (OCT)-based methods for quantifying drusen progression and drusen volume. Polarization-sensitive OCT is the most promising of these approaches and will be used to quantify drusen area and volume in the present study.

TYPE OF STUDY - Observational

NUMBER OF PATIENTS TO BE ENROLLED - 300

STUDY SITE - Medical University of Vienna, Vienna, Austria

PRINCIPAL INVESTIGATOR - Stefan Sacu, MD Medical University of Vienna

CONTACT - Gerhard Garhofer, MD
００４３１４０４００２９８１

gerhard.garhoefer@meduniwien.ac.at
Stefan Sacu, MD
stefan.sacu@meduniwien.ac.at

LENGTH OF STUDY - START DATE - March 2014
- END DATE - January 2018

PROCEDURE - Not provided

DETAILED DESCRIPTION -

Drusen area and volume will be measured using polarization sensitive OCT

Visual Acuity and Refraction

Choroidal blood flow

Macular pigment optical density

****
****
****
****
****
****

NOTES

The eye is an attractive target for gene therapy for the following reasons:

1. It is one of the few immunologically privileged sites in the body. Gene vectors are unlikely to a cause a systemic immune response.

2. The eye has a small, defined volume. Small amounts of viral vectors may achieve a therapeutic benefit, while minimizing the risk of systemic toxicity.

3. The effects of locally administered ocular treatments can be easily monitored for efficacy and safety.

In 2008, 3 research groups, two in the U.S. and one in the UK, reported success in RPE65-associated LCA using the adeno-associated viral (AAV2) vector. Patients recovered functional vision without significant side-effects. But, the improvement lasted for approximately 3 years as further photoreceptor degeneration continued to advance in the treated retinas at the same rate as the untreated.

Adeno-associated viruses (AAV) are non-pathogenic small viruses with one strand of DNA from the parvovirus family. AAV vectors have a low risk of mutagenesis and have a high rate of successful insertion of genetic material into specific sites.

AAV-mediated gene therapy only works if there are still target cells remaining. Going forward, treatment may consist of a vector containing the specific gene for correcting the disease, and a second viral vector containing complementary DNA for neuro-protection. In this manner, the genetic defect may be corrected, while a cell-protective, or inhibition of a cell-death pathway also occurs. Conceptually it is better to intervene early, before significant degeneration has occurred.

The treatment of neovascular or "wet" AMD requires the frequent injection of medications. Local gene transfer offers the possibility of sustained drug delivery to the retina. Pre-clinical testing in animal models suggests that the intravitreal injection of a gene product, AAV2-sFLT01, can inhibit neovascular activity for a sustained period of time.

Another avenue for activity is the treatment of the Complement pathway, which mediates the inflammatory component of AMD. Hemera Bioscience is testing HMR59, which is an AAV2 vector that expresses soluble CD59. CD59 is a naturally occurring protein that protects cells from complement damage. Testing in a neovascularization mouse model demonstrated that the prior intravitreal injection of HMR59 inhibited the formation of choroidal neovascular membranes by 56%.

```
******************************
******************************
****************
******************************
******************************
****************
```

www.ingramcontent.com/pod-product-compliance
Lightning Source LLC
Chambersburg PA
CBHW031434210526
45464CB00005B/2202